I0438006

FAITH AND HEALING

REV. FR. JOSEPH K. BILL, V.C.

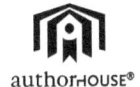

authorHOUSE®

AuthorHouse™
1663 Liberty Drive
Bloomington, IN 47403
www.authorhouse.com
Phone: 1-800-839-8640

Published by AuthorHouse   12/28/2012

ISBN: 978-1-4343-9108-7 (sc)
ISBN: 978-1-4343-9105-6 (e)

First and second editions published 2001 and 2006, respectively, by Goodnews Media Centre, Palarivattom, Kochi, Kerala, India, and edited by Sabu Jose.
This USA edition published 2008 at the personal request and authorization of Fr. Joseph K. Bill, V.C., by Fr. Joseph K. Bill Ministries, Inc., 3128 Leyland Trail, Woodbury, MN 55125 USA, on the Internet at www.FrBillUSA.net.

A Tribute to late Rev. Fr. Joseph K. Bill

We were so familiar with his simple and down to earth teachings of catholic faith. He often said "Jesus suffered for us and died on the cross for us. So this love must be repaid. That is why we have decided to follow Jesus Christ." He was so convinced of this in his life that he was working day and night to fulfill the same in his own life. He used to say that God repaired his heart about 32 years back when he had his first heart attack, just to spread the love and forgiveness of Jesus to every nook and corner of this world. The Almighty called him back to take rest in His presence after 50 years of sincere and faithful service as a Priest.

Fr. Joseph Kuruppamparambil, Fr. Bill for short, was born on Feb 23, 1928 as the fourth son of Xavier and Anna at Thottakam, Vaikom, Kerala, India. He joined the Vincentian Congregation, a Catholic Religious Organization founded in Kerala, South India, made his first profession on May 22, 1952, final profession on January 5, 1956 and was ordained a priest on October 12,

1958 by His Eminence, late Joseph Cardinal Parekkattil, the then archbishop of Ernakulam Archdiocese.

Fr. Joseph Kuruppamparambil VC joined St. Vincent's minor seminary in 1948. He was one of the 10 seminarians of the first batch. Even before he was admitted in the seminary, while he was in the high school classes, he started a project of spreading anti-Communist literature called INTEC, which indeed was very effective in the long run. In the seminary, a group of Brothers joined together under the leadership of Brother Joseph with the idea of spreading certain devotional practices so as to foster genuine piety among the seminarians especially devotion to Blessed Virgin Mary.

Soon after his Ordination, he involved himself headlong in man various activities both spiritual and temporal, such as parish works, and procurator ship of our Generalate. He initiated so many social activities wherever he worked. Total involvement was his characteristic note. Throughout his life he was very optimistic, always cheerful, never depressed, even in very trying circumstances. He never showed a grim face even in very tough situations he had to encounter several times in life. He was responsible for starting schools under the auspices of our congregation especially English Medium Schools, which were very rare in the state at that time. He was never discouraged or lost hope.

Fr. Bill was very adventurous and such a spirit was visible wherever he was appointed and what ever he did. His initiative, imagination, originality, his capacity to captivate hearts and minds, his ever-smiling face and every diplomatic step he took, reveal his colorful personality and unique leadership qualities. There are many orphanages and schools for the poor to his credit and initiative. It was not his nature to do things half way. He used to be totally immersed in whatever he did. Dynamism in its most intense form had been always noted in him. Even when he had been attached to many offices in each house, he was preoccupied and engaged in preaching Popular Mission retreats and later Charismatic Retreats.

He was in the Novitiate when the first popular mission retreat of our congregation was conducted. It was in 1951. He was an active participant in it and settled some adventurous cases that disrupted the unity of families. Soon after his Ordination, he jumped headlong in organizing Popular Missions and conducting effectively various items of the Mission, which were which were all novel to the faithful. It was his originality and hard work that added new items and nuances to the customary practices that projected the great new Renewal Program, which was the Popular Mission. So we can say that he is one of the pioneers of the Popular Mission and to a great extent the one who paved way to its growth and spread of it throughout the length and breadth of the country.

Clarity, effectiveness and practicality marked his preaching always. His commanding personality, his musical trend always captured the attention of the audience in great numbers. He was always a crowd-puller, not only in India, but also all over the world. So many reports of total cure of the personality were coming to us. He was effectively diplomatic in his relationships with others. He was always generous to others. He practiced the principle of St. Paul that charity covers a multitude of sins. There are occasions when persons duped him in view of his generosity. He never kept any grudge against any body. Whenever he met even his bitterest enemies, he welcomed them as close friends smiling and in a considerate mood. That is why he used to say, "Unless we forgive from our hearts our Heavenly Father will not forgive the multitude of our sins. We will have to remain in purgatory until the last bit of our sins is removed. This is the importance of forgiveness in our lives. Do not forget it." We cannot forget his sterling qualities and what he did for the Vincentian Congregation especially for the African Mission and individuals in difficulties - spiritual, mental and material.

It was in 1992 that he came to the East African Mission of the Vincentian Congregation with lots of enthusiasm to preach the Good News to the people in East Africa. His first attempt in Tanzania transformed many unbelievers into true apostles of Jesus. Very soon news about this zealous Vincentian Missionary spread far and wide in the whole African Continent. His retreats attracted people in large numbers. People, irrespective of faith, nationality and color flocked to his preaching sessions. Meanwhile, he started getting requests from all over the world to conduct healing services. Consequently, he became an international preacher of great reputation within a short time. Bundles of passports and the retreat schedule he always carried will make one understand just how busy he was as a true messenger of Jesus' love and forgiveness.

The future generation would remember him as a legendary figure. In spite of his human limitations and failures, he always remained a focus of attention. Clarity of his vision, insight, his meticulous planning, boundless confidence, zeal, practicality, dynamism, leadership qualities perhaps unparalleled his capacity to remain close to all those he came across, his simple life style, his ambition to do things ordinarily unattainable for the common man. A person who met him for the first time will definitely get himself engrossed in the mesmerizing personality. He was immersed in his preaching ministry so much so he had no time for any other entertainment except sharing the word of God.

His simple life style of wearing the priestly habit all throughout his life, whether at home or abroad elicited surprise as well as high respect from his on lookers. He never cared for his personal comforts. Hours and hours he spent for preaching, standing on his feet, causing edema in his feet. The word impossible was never in his dictionary. This year was his Sacerdotal Golden Jubilee. He did not see 50th anniversary of his Priestly Ordination. A few months before his golden jubilee in October, his Heavenly Father called him home. He had just celebrated his 80th birthday in February. At a time when it was the least expected, the drop-scene of his life drama took place and all those who loved him mourn for his unexpected departure to attain his eternal life.

May his soul rest in peace.

Fr. Vincent Rathappillil

(Regional Superior)

ABOUT THE AUTHOR

Fr. Bill went to be with the Lord on March 14, 2008, having celebrated his 80th birthday the previous month, and anticipating celebrating the 50th anniversary of his ordination later in 2008. Having preached all day (as was usual 365 days a year with Father), he felt some pain in the evening, and then died in the arms of his disciple and successor, Fr. Anthony, while on the way to the hospital. The heart Jesus re-created for Fr. Bill in 1976, he had now worn out with apostolic labors, and now his Heavenly Father called him home. "Well done, good and faithful servant! Enter into the joy of your Lord!"

Originally from Kerala, India, Fr. Joseph K. Bill, V.C. (Vincentian Congregation) had been a missionary in East Africa beginning in 1992, until his death. He preached retreats and popular missions not only in India and East Africa, but all over Europe, the United States, Canada, and Korea. He gave the message of the Good News to bishops, priests and lay people, and through his ministry the Lord Jesus brought numerous healing – spiritual, mental/emotional and physical – to thousands. In Africa he once gave a week's retreat to a million people at once.

Regularly his missions and retreats numbered in the thousands and required outdoor stadiums.

Beloved of all who knew him, Fr. Bill radiated the Love of Jesus so powerfully that even hardened people felt loved. With his simple stories he conveyed the truths of the Bible and taught the eternal faith of the Catholic Church In his prayer for healing, deliverance and exorcism, and absolute confidence in God, he demonstrated the kind of absolute faith and trust in Jesus who cannot lie that he always spoke of. His schedule was booked year round because his love for God's children would not let him rest. Even in the last year of his life, he continued to say, "I do not want to rest. I want to bring Jesus to the people!" The source of his nourishment was daily Holy Mass which he prayed devoutly, and several hours a day in prayer, always rising hours before dawn to first spend time with his God before anything else.

Fr. Bill is buried at the Miraculous Medal Shrine at the Vincentian Centre in Entebbe, Uganda, where he had always desired to be buried because of his great love for the East African people.

Fr. Bill often said he would never lie still, not even in Heaven. While on earth, he so lovingly spoke of Jesus face to face with us. Now we believe he is lovingly speaking face to face with Jesus about us, his children still on earth. Fr. Joseph K. Bill, pray for us.

CHAPTER 1
THE HEALING TOUCH

The paths of Jerusalem were crowded. People were swarming around Jesus who was traveling through the city of Jerusalem. No one knew from where but a timid woman pushed herself through the thickly packed crowd. She was all wrapped in clothing. She was embarrassed and deeply anxious. But there was something fiery in her. Something like a burning desire – a desire to get healing. For she had been suffering from hemorrhages for the past 12 years.

Through the pressing crowd she approached Jesus. She had tremendous faith. She believed that she would indeed be healed if only she touched the mantle of Jesus. And she touched. Instantly she was healed!

Even Jesus was astounded. He felt that healing power flow out of Him. He turned and asked, "Who touched me?" Peter the disciple wondered; for he has been seeing hundreds of people pushing Jesus from all sides. It would be better to ask, "Who is not touching me?"! But Jesus insisted that someone had really touched Him. He kept on asking, "Who touched me?" Then the woman who had received healing timidly came forward and said, "Master, it was I who touched you." Jesus told her, "Your faith has healed you!" (Lk. 8:43-48)

This is one of the most powerful pictures of faith healing presented in the Scriptures. It is exactly a healing by faith. Let us now examine the process once again. Take note that Jesus recognizes the gush of power from Him only when the power has gone out. There were hundreds of touches. But He feels something extraordinary in a particular touch because behind that touch there was the strength of faith. That is the touch of faith. No other touch in the crowd was able to bring out that power. Moreover, the woman knew that a mere touch on the edge of the cloak of Jesus would heal her. That is faith. That is the power of faith!

The Holy Scriptures is abounding in examples of persons who gained healing from God by the virtue of their faith.

My Healing

Now, let me share with you my own experiences with faith and healing. I am a Vincentian priest. As you know, a charism of our congregation is serving the poor. So, as priest, naturally I engaged myself with taking care of an orphanage. Even at that time I had love for Jesus. I did my services for Jesus' sake. Yet there was something lacking in me. At that time I did not have the absolute faith that I have now. I was like any other Catholic in the world.

One day, as I was praying during the Holy Mass, I fell down unconscious. I was in the unconscious state for three days. My friends and relatives thought that I was going to die. So they were ardently praying for me. On the fourth day I got back my consciousness. The doctor said to me, "You are in a very critical state. You have already had two heart attacks. The third one would be fatal."

While I was under a prescribed strict rest I heard that there was a Charismatic retreat about to be conducted for priests and bishops. Although I hated the Charismatic way in those days, I decided to go to the retreat because I wanted to be healed. At that time my faith was not as strong as it is now. Still, because of my ardent desire to be healed, I went to the retreat.

There were 163 priests and two bishops attending the retreat. As part of the retreat there was a healing service. It was one bishop who prayed over me. He asked me what I wanted to be prayed for in particular. I said that I wanted to be healed. I had decided that if I were to be healed I would do something very good for Jesus Christ. The bishop prayed over me. Then I saw Jesus in flesh and blood standing before me. Jesus touched me. And I was completely healed!

The next day the result of the laboratory test proved the miraculous. There was not the least sign of a heart attack! The doctor could not believe it. He said that it was impossible in the sight of the medical science. He sent for a repeat test. Then he asked how it all happened. I said, "The God who created me has the power to heal me. The God who has created my heart has the ability to give me a new heart!" The result of the second test confirmed the first result. The doctor admitted that it was a miraculous cure. It was a divine healing. That was how God taught me to believe – to believe absolutely and completely.

THE GOD WHO CREATED YOU

Once a man was riding in a new Ford car. On the way the car broke down. The man got down and began to examine the car. But neither he nor his driver could find out what has happened to the car. As they were standing, a man came along their way. Seeing a car being halted on the way and the perplexed passengers, the man stopped his car. He asked them what had happened. They revealed their dilemma. The newcomer opened the hood of the car, connected a small piece of wire, got into the car and started it with ease. The owner of the car was surprised. They had been toiling for hours with no success. But this man had mended the car within seconds. He asked him, "Who are you?" "I am Mr. Henry Ford." He was the man who built the car. He knew every detail of the car he made.

In the same way God knows exactly where our problem lies. He has created us. He has created our soul, our mind and our body. If He has created them He has indeed the power to re-create them. God can re-create your damaged heart, your liver, your kidney, your lungs, your pancreas and every part of your body. Because He is the Author of our body, He can repair the parts of our body even without the aid of medicines. It is God who gives the healing power to the medicines themselves. Faith is all we need. Faith in the absolute power of God.

MY FAITH EXPERIENCES

After my healing I returned to my monastery and told my superior that I wanted to preach about Jesus Christ who has healed me. The superior had doubts. He told me that I would die if I tire myself. I believed in Jesus and I said that I was ready to climb up a huge hill to prove my healing. It was a hill in Kerala called Malayatoor. I took with me a boy as a companion and climbed that hill. Then my superior was convinced and allowed me to go out preaching.

My faith was growing. Then I wanted to study about faith healing. For that I went to Duquesne University in Pittsburg in America. One day while I was praying with Charismatic people in a church of Boston, a paralyzed man was brought to our midst. They asked me to pray over the man. So I place my hands on his head and prayed over him. As I was praying over him, Jesus told me in my heart, "Tell him to get up and walk." I did not doubt. I knew that Jesus was God and that He would never tell a lie. I told the paralyzed man to get up and walk. Instantly, the man got up and walked. Everybody was astounded. Even I was shocked. I did not expect so much. It was a clear miracle of God.

That incident strengthened my faith. The same Jesus Who walked along the shore of Galilee, Who passed through the streets of Judea healing the sick, is alive here and now! He can heal you! What He demands from you is faith. You need nothing but a complete trust in God's power. "If you believe, you shall see the glory of God!" (Jn. 11:40.)

JESUS THE HEALER

Centuries before the birth of Christ, Isaiah had prophesied, "We are healed by his infirmities." (Is. 53:5) Jesus was wounded for our iniquities. He has taken up our wounds upon Himself. Jesus died for our sake. It is Jesus Who heals. He is the "Wounded Healer." Mathew the Evangelist remarks when Jesus heals the sick., "He cast out demons by the Word and healed all the sick. The prophecy of Isaiah, 'He took our weaknesses and carried our infirmities' thus became true." (Mt. 8:16-17)

HEALING IS THE LOVE OF GOD

Healing is the love of God. It is God's love taking our infirmities upon Him-self. God the Father sends His own

Son to the world in order to save mankind. To take away the sufferings and sicknesses of mankind that are caused by the sin of man. Jesus, the Son of God comes to the world, takes upon Himself all our wounds and sicknesses, and dies on the cross. This is the great love of God. Every healing is God's love manifested.

It is exactly as the story of the prodigal son in the Gospel. He loses everything: his health, his wealth his self esteem, and so on. But the loving father rehabilitates him when he comes back. The father in the story is the representative of God the Father. God gives back everything to the sinner who turns back to Him. Yes, it is the love of God that heals.

CHAPTER 2
SIN - THE SOURCE OF ALL SUFFERINGS

We know that today's world is full of agonies and sufferings. We hear about war. Our age has witnessed many disastrous wars. Terrible and devastating natural calamities earthquakes, Tsunami, Hurricane Katrina, Rita and so on constantly hit the world. Homicides are rampant. Suicides, abortions! Life is valued least. The psychological life of man has lost its balance. Depression has taken over the reins of the human mind.

Medical science has advanced so much. We have found new medicines. But still even newer sicknesses arise. Cancer, Aids, Anthrax. Man is in the vicious circle of illnesses. The more medicines are invented, the more illnesses are spreading. Pain and sufferings are abounding. And we ask God: "Why it is so?"

Why Suffering?

Man has always sought for the reason for the sufferings of mankind. Why is there pain? Why is there sickness? Why sorrow? Different people have found different answers. Several philosophers and thinkers have put forth various arguments and theories.

Buddha says that desire is the cause of suffering. But if we are going to negate every desire, what about the desire for good? If desire is the cause of suffering, how did suffering and pain come into the universe for the first time?

The Scriptures say that God saw that everything was good when He created the universe. The life of man was joyful. He was in peace with the nature and other living beings. There was an abiding harmony among man, the universe and God. Then how did he lose that harmony and balance?

The book of Genesis has the story of the Paradise lost. The sin of man broke the harmony between God, man and the universe. Man disobeyed God. He disbelieved the Word of God. God had told Adam and Eve not to eat from the tree from the center of the Garden of Eden. But the man and his wife believed Satan rather than God. They disbelieved God. That was the sin of man. Thus man was out of the Paradise. "Cursed be the ground because of you. In toil you shall eat of it all the days in your life. Thorns and thistles it shall bring forth for you. And you shall eat the plants of the field. By the sweat of your face you shall eat bread until you return to the ground. For it is out of it you were taken. You are dust, and to dust you shall return." (Gen. 3:17-19) Sufferings came into the world as the natural result of the sin of man.

Today medical science has found out that evil deeds breed evil waves into world. In Japan, some scientists have found out that the deeds of man generate positive and negative waves according to the good and bad acts of man respectively. Negative waves cause hatred and suffering. They cause sicknesses. The positive waves produce peace and love. According to them there are four kinds of positive waves. They have named it alpha, beta, theta and delta. These positive waves repel the negative waves that cause illnesses and hatred. The medical experts say that a kind of soothing and curing oil is produced by our love when we love. In the same way a sort of poisonous oil is produced by hatred. This poisonous oil causes sickness.

Sin Causes Sickness

The gospel of St. Mathew has a beautiful account of a healing taking place as a result of one's sins been forgiven by Jesus.

"And just then some people were carrying a paralyzed man lying on a bed. . . . When Jesus saw their faith, He said to the paralytic, 'Take heart, son; your sins are forgiven.' Then some of the scribes said to themselves. 'This man is blaspheming.' But Jesus, perceiving their thoughts, said, 'Why do you think evil in your hearts?

For which is easier, to say, "Your sins are forgiven," or to say, "Stand up and walk"? But so that you may know that the Son of Man has authority on earth to forgive sins,' He then said to the paralytic, 'Stand up! Take your bed and go to your home.' And he stood up, and went to his home.'" (Mt. 9:2-7)

Here, Jesus clearly states that the sin of the paralytic man has been a great impediment to receive healing. Before healing the man, Jesus takes away the bondage of sin that has kept him under its slavery.

At another instance, we can see Jesus telling a man whom he had healed at the pool of Bethesda, "See, you have been made well! Do not sin anymore, so that nothing worse happens to you." (Jn. 5:14)

There are several instances in the Bible, which clearly state that sin can be the cause of sicknesses. Even today many sicknesses are caused by the sin of man. Aids spread in the world because of the licentious sexual culture of the world. When man turns away from God and indulge in Godless and evil activities, his body and mind would rebel against man. The nature will rebel against man.

In my life I have come across several incidents in which man is suffering because of his past sins. I knew a man utterly ruined in his old age suffering terribly from serious illness. When I met him, he confessed to me that in his youth he had brutally persecuted a poor family. The members of the poor family did not take revenge upon him. But the impact of his own sin and the unavoidable justice of God abandoned him to suffering and illnesses.

It does not mean that every sickness is caused by sin. There can be other physical reasons for one's illness. There can be salvific sufferings and sicknesses as St. Therese of Liseaux had. But the suffering and illnesses of mankind as a whole is the result of sin. Sickness is the lack of perfection. Something is wanting to the body. Something has decayed within the body. This happens due to sin. Sin takes away the grace of God from man. It is the grace and the presence of God that make man whole. When God is lost, the completeness is lost; fullness is lost.

WHO CAN HEAL YOU?

Who can heal the illnesses of the world? The one who has taken way the sin of the world! (Jn. 1:20) Jesus Christ, the Savior of the world. It is about this Jesus that prophet Isaiah proclaimed, "Surely he has borne our infirmities and carried our diseases. . . . He was wounded for our transgressions, crushed for our iniquities; upon him was the punishment that made us whole, and by his bruises we are healed." (Is. 53:4-5)

It is true that the medical experts and doctors can treat you and give you medicines. But the healing comes from God. If God does not heal the treatment of doctor is in vain. Our healing is bought by the blood of Jesus Christ. The Word of God says, "For neither herb nor poultice cured them, but it was Your word, O Lord, that heals all people." (Wis. 16:12)

Healing by Faith

As the Bible says, all healing comes from God. God can use the medicines and the skill of the doctors to heal a person. At the same time He can do it without anybody's mediation - without the aid of medicine. That is faith-healing. It is miraculous healing. The only thing God demands from us in order to receive healing is faith. Faith and trust in God's love and power.

CHAPTER 3
FAITH IN GOD

WHAT IS FAITH?

After the sin of Adam, God kept his promise of the advent of the Savior alive through prophecies. He spoke through the prophets through centuries. Through them He was manifesting His will to mankind. Finally, God revealed Himself to the world through His only Son, Jesus Christ. Jesus Christ is the fullness of revelation. He came into the world, took birth as the Son of Mary, preached the word, healed the sick, forgave sinners, suffered and died on the cross. As the Apostle says, "In the earlier times, God spoke through the prophets, and finally He spoke through His own Son." (Heb. 1:1) Faith is the response of man to this revelation of God. It is the wholehearted and humble acceptance of that truth and mystery.

After the resurrection of Jesus, when he appeared to his disciples, Thomas, the apostle, was not there. And when the other apostles told him that they had seen Jesus, Thomas doubted. He argued that he would never believe it unless he sees Jesus directly and put his finger into His wounds. Then Jesus appeared another time. This time, Thomas was also present. Jesus said to Thomas, "Put your fingers here and see My hands. Reach out your hand and put it in My side . . . Blessed are those who have not seen and yet come to believe!" (Jn. 20:27-29)

These words of Jesus are the basis of Christian faith. Believing without seeing. We have not seen Jesus walking in our streets. If we believe still, we are blessed. It is the conviction that unseen things exist and that we will inherit what we hope for.

The Faith of Abraham

Abraham is the father of the faithful. When God called Abraham for the first time, he did not know the true God. But once he came to know the true God, Yahweh, he never doubted God. God asked him to leave back the land of his ancestors and his own people, and to go to an alien land. Abraham obeyed God without any doubt. He had absolute faith in God.

"By faith Abraham obeyed when he was called to set out for a place that he was to receive as an inheritance. And he set out, not knowing where he was going. By faith he stayed for a time in the land he had been promised, as in a foreign land. . . . By faith he received the power of procreation, even though he was too old, and Sarah herself was barren, because he considered Him faithful who had promised. Therefore from one person, and this one as good as dead, descendants were born, 'as many as the stars of heaven and as innumerable grains of sand by the seashore'" (Heb. 11:8-12)

It was at a time when there was the least possibility for Abraham and Sarah of having a son, that God promised them a son. By normal reason it would have seemed impossible. Yet, Abraham believed the word of God. And he received the reward. He begot a son in his late old age. Years later, when his beloved son Isaac was growing up, God asked Abraham to sacrifice his son. This would have been utterly painful for Abraham. God is asking his only son! But by faith Abraham obeyed.

"By faith Abraham, when put to the test, offered up Isaac. He who had received the promises was ready to offer up his only son, of whom he had been told, 'It is through Isaac that descendants shall be named for you.' He considered the fact that God is able to raise someone from the dead and, figuratively speaking, he did receive him back." (Heb. 11:17-19) That is how Abraham became the Father of the faithful.

FAITH OF THE FATHERS OF THE OLD TESTAMENT

All the ancient fathers in the Old Testament are men of faith. They lived by faith. They obeyed whatever God had commanded them. Even though they did not see God they believed in Him and obeyed Him.

"By faith Isaac invoked blessings for the future on Jacob and Esau. By faith Jacob, when dying, blessed each of the sons of Joseph, 'bowing in worship over the top of his staff.' By faith Joseph, at the end of his life, made mention of the exodus of the Israelites and gave instructions about his burial. By faith Moses was hidden by his parents for three months after his birth, because they saw that the child was beautiful; and they were not afraid of the king's edict. By faith Moses, when grown up, refused to be called a son of Pharaoh's daughter, choosing rather to share ill-treatment with the people of God rather than to enjoy the fleeting pleasures of sin. He considered abuse suffered for the Christ to be greater wealth than the treasures of Egypt, for he was looking ahead to the reward. By faith he left Egypt, unafraid of the king's anger. For he perceived as though he saw the invisible." (Heb. 11:23-27)

Besides these fathers, there is a chain of faithful people who kept their faith in God: Samson, Gideon, David, and so on. David defeated the giant Goliath by faith. In human standards, Goliath, the giant Philistine, was much stronger than David who was only a shepherd boy. But David who believed in the Almighty God took up the challenge of the Philistine. With a few pebbles he defeated and killed the giant. Let us see the account of the Scriptures: "David said to the Philistine, 'You come to me with sword and spear and javelin, but I come to you in the name of the Lord of hosts, the God of the armies of Israel, whom you have defied. This very day the Lord will deliver you into my hand, and I will strike you down and cut off your head; and I will give the dead bodies of the Philistine army this very day to the birds of the air and to the wild animals of the earth, so that all the animals of the earth may know that there is a God in Israel!'" (I Sam. 17:45-46)

HEROIC FAITH OF A JEWISH MOTHER AND HER SONS

In the Old Testament, in book of Maccabees, there is an inspiring incident depicted of a heroic mother and her seven sons. It was during the reign of the pagan ruler Antiochus. He insisted that all the Jewish people must eat the flesh of swine, which was forbidden to them. Many profaned themselves by eating the forbidden flesh. But there was a faithful mother and her seven sons. They were brought before the king. But all of them refused to eat the forbidden flesh, because they did not want to offend the Lord by violating His commandments. The king threatened them and tortured them. But they kept their faith. She encouraged her sons by these words, "I do not know how you came into being in my womb. It was not I who gave you breath, nor I who set in order the elements within each of you. Therefore, the Creator of the world, who shaped the beginning of humankind and devised the origin of all things, will in His mercy give life and breath back to you again, since you now forget yourselves for the sake of the laws." (2 Mc. 7:22-23). Thus all her sons underwent heroic martyrdom for the sake of faith.

19

Faith in the New Testament

The New Testament is the age of the fullness of revelation and faith. More faith is demanded from mankind to receive and accept the new revelation of Jesus Christ. There are many models of faith in the New Testament.

Faith of Mary

Mary, the mother of Jesus, is the foremost example of faith in the New Testament. Mary was a virgin who had decided to remain a virgin all through her life when the angel of the Lord appeared to her announcing the birth of the Savior. Naturally she could have disbelieved the word of God like Zechariah. Any human being would naturally doubt the announcement that a virgin would conceive without the assistance of a man. Mary naturally expressed her question. But the greatness of Mary's faith lies in her surrender when he promises the work of the Holy Spirit in the conception. She says, "Behold the Handmaid of the Lord. Let it be done according to your word." (Lk. 1:38) She believes the impossible! It was because she believed that she received the privilege to become the mother of the Lord.

Mary could have had other reasons to resist the promise of God. Her Jewish society, which never tolerates any illegal childbirth, would condemn Mary to death, punishment for having conceived before marriage. She was in fact in danger. But she put her complete trust in God. She believed that the God in whom she trusted would certainly take care of her.

The Faith of the Centurion

"I tell you, not even in Israel have I found such faith!" These are the words with which Jesus gives testimony to the faith of a pagan centurion. The evangelist Luke narrates the event: "Once as Jesus entered Capernaum, a centurion there had a slave whom he valued highly, and who was ill and close to death. When he heard about Jesus, he sent some Jewish elders to him, asking him to come and heal his slave. When they came to Jesus, they appealed to him earnestly, saying, 'He is worthy of having you do this for him, for he loves our people, and it is he who built our synagogue for us.' And Jesus went with them. But when He was not far from the house, the centurion sent friends to say to Him, 'Lord, do not trouble yourself, for I am not worthy to have You come under my roof. Therefore I did not consider myself worthy to come to You; but only speak the word, and let my servant be healed. For I also am a man set under authority, with soldiers under me, and I say to one, "Go," and he goes, and to another, "Come," and he comes, and to the slave, "Do this," and he does it.' When Jesus heard this He was amazed at him, and turning to the crowd that followed Him, He said, 'I tell you, not even in Israel have I found such faith!'" (Lk. 7:2-9)

The Faith of the Canaanite Woman

Another great example of faith is the Canaanite woman whose faith Jesus praised. This woman was after Jesus begging for the cure of her daughter who had been tormented by a demon. But Jesus blatantly ignored her request. But the woman kept on pleading to Jesus. Then Jesus turned to her and said, "I was sent only to the lost sheep of the house of Israel." But she came and knelt before him, saying, "Lord, help me." He answered "it is not fair to take the children's food and throw it to the dogs." She said, "Yes, Lord, yet even the dogs eat the crumbs that fall from their master's table." Then Jesus answered her, "Woman, your faith is great! Let it be done for you as you wish."

Take note that Jesus was apparently insulting her by degrading her to status of dogs. It was to test her faith that He did so. But her faith was great. Her faith surprised even Jesus.

Faith of the Early Christians and Martyrs

Martyrdom for Christ actually begins from St. John the Baptist. He stood for the truth and justice of God. He accused the illegal relationship of King Herod and Herodias. Because of his faith, he resisted and overcame all threats of the king and his concubine. But the revengeful Herodias influenced the King through the dance of her daughter Salome, and had John the Baptist beheaded.

Martyrdom of St. Stephan

The first martyr for Jesus Christ in history was St. Stephen. St. Luke writes about St. Stephan in the Acts of the Apostles. "Stephen, full of grace and power, did great wonders and signs among the people." (Acts 6:8) He was a fearless follower of Christ. He preached Christ. This infuriated the Jews and they decided to stone him to death. "When they heard these things, they became enraged and ground their teeth at Stephen. But filled with the Holy Spirit, he gazed into heaven and saw the glory of God and Jesus standing at the right hand of God. 'Look,' he said, 'I see the heavens opened and the Son of Man standing at the right hand of God!' But they covered their ears, and with a loud shout all rushed together against him. Then they dragged him out of the city and began to stone him; and the witnesses laid their costs at the feet of a young man named Saul. While they were stoning Stephen, he prayed, 'Lord Jesus, receive my spirit.' Then he knelt down and cried out in a loud voice, 'Lord, do not hold this sin against them.' When he had said this, he died." (Acts 7:54-60)

The Christians Who Died for the Faith

Following the martyrdom of St. Stephen, there was a long chain of martyrs through the centuries. There arose vehement persecution of the Church by the Roman emperors such as Nero and Diocletian. Thousands of

Christians were killed. In those days the Christian had flaming faith. They laid down their lives courageously. Young girls like St. Agnes, St. Agatha, and St. Cecilia embraced martyrdom. Holy and courageous bishops like St. Ignatius of Antioch and St. Poly-carp of Smyrna laid down their lives for Christ. The persecution of the Church lasted for about three centuries. Thousands and thousands of Christians shed their blood for their faith in Jesus during this period. As someone said, "The blood of the martyrs became the manure for the growth of the Catholic Church."

WE NEED FAITH

There are people in today's world who argue that faith is unnecessary. They believe only in the scientific truths proved in laboratories. But there are many things that cannot be proved in laboratories. For example, love. I cannot show you my love the way I show you a flower. I can express my love though my words and actions. I cannot see wind. But I can experience wind. I believe that I am the son or daughter of so and so because my mother has told me so. I believe my mother. In every day life we believe a lot of things. We do not ask for proof for anything and everything in our daily life. Friendship and family life depends upon mutual faith. Without faith there is no possibility of relationship. The reason for all the calamities, war and dissensions in the world is the absence of faith.

We need not only this kind of human faith. Human faith is essential to live on in this world, but supernatural faith is essential to inherit eternal life. Faith, hope and love are the eternal virtues. Faith is the trustful longing for the things that we have not yet seen, which we will inherit in the future. We need this supernatural faith in order to attain healing. Faith is the essential pre-requisite for faith-healing.

Chapter 4
FAITH HEALING IN THE SCRIPTURES

The Holy Bible says, "Neither herb nor poultice cured them, but it was your word, O Lord, that heals all people." (Wis. 16:12) We are dealing with healing by the power of God through faith. The God who created you from nothingness can heal you without the aid of medical science and doctors. In the first chapter of this book, I had narrated the way I received a miraculous cure, and my experience of curing a paralyzed man in the church in Boston. I have witnesses hundreds and hundreds of such cases in my ministry. Jesus is God. So He will never say a lie. Jesus has promised, "They will lay their hands on the sick, and they will recover." (Mk. 16:18)

Healing in the Old Testament

In the book of Kings we see the prophet Elijah reviving the life of the son of the widow of Zarephath. It is narrated, "After this, the son of the woman, the mistress of the house, became ill. His illness was so severe that there was no breath left in him. She then said to Elijah, 'What have you against me, O man of God? You have come to me to bring my sin to remembrance and to cause the death of my son!' But he said to her, 'Give me your son.' He took him from her bosom, carried him up into the upper chamber where he was lodging, and laid him on his own bed. He cried out to the Lord, 'O Lord my God, have you brought calamity even upon the widow with whom I am staying, by killing her son?' Then he stretched himself upon the child three times, and cried out to the Lord, 'O Lord my God, let this child's life come into him again.' The Lord listened to the voice of Elijah. The life of the child came into him again, and he revived." (I Kings 17:17:22)

Another great incident of miraculous healing is the healing of Namaan by the prophet Elisha. The Bible writes, "Naman, commander of the army of the king of Aram, was a great man in his favor with his master, because by him the Lord has given victory of Aram. The man, though a mighty warrior, suffered from leprosy." (2 Kings 5:1) He heard about Ellsha, the man of God who was in Israel, and sent word to him. Elisha asked him to wash himself in the river Jordan. "But Namaan became angry and went away saying, 'I thought that for me he would surely come out, and stand and call on the name of the Lord his God, and would wave his hand over the spot, and cure the leprosy. Are not Abana and Phropar the rivers of Damascus better than all the waters of Israel? Could I not wash in them, and be clean?' He turned and went away in a rage. But his servants approached and said to him, 'Father, if the prophet had commanded you to do something difficult, would you not have done it? How much more, when all he said to you was, "Wash, and be clean"? So he went down and immersed himself seven times in the Jordan, according to the word of the man of God. His flesh was restored like the flesh of a young boy, and he was clean." (2 Kings 5:11-14)

Here are the two major incidents of healing in the Old Testament. Elijah and Elisha were great prophets of God. God had given them power of heal because of their profound faith and dedication to the will of God.

King Hezekiah's Illness and Healing

Another remarkable incident in the Old Testament is the healing of Hezekiah, the King of Judah. This incident clearly depicts how God hears man's prayer and heals him.

"In those days Hezekiah became sick and was at the point of death. The prophet Isaiah, son of Amoz came to him, and said to him, 'Thus says the Lord: set your house in order, for you shall die; you shall not recover.' Then Hezekiah turned his face to the wall and prayed to the Lord, 'Remember now, O Lord, I implore you, how have I walked before You in faithfulness with a wide heart, and have done what is good in Your sight.' Hezekiah wept bitterly. Before Isaiah had gone out of the middle court the word of the Lord came to him, 'Turn back, and say to

Hezekiah, prince of My people, 'Thus says the Lord, the God of your ancestor David: I have heard your prayer, I have seen your tears. Indeed, I will heal you. On the third day you shall go up to the house of the Lord. I will add fifteen years to your life." (2 Kings 20:1-7)

And as God had promised, Hezekiah was healed, and he lived for fifteen more years.

JESUS AND HEALING

If we analyze the Gospels, we will be able to see that among the miracles done by Jesus, the healing of the sick was prominent. Jesus, when revealing himself to the people gathered in the synagogue announces, "The spirit of the Lord is upon me, because he has anointed me to bring good news to the poor. He has sent me to proclaim release to the captives and recovery of sight to the blind, to let the oppressed go free, to proclaim the year of the Lord's favor." (Lk. 4:18-19)

When Jesus proclaimed that He was anointed to "recover the sight of the blind", to let the oppressed go free" etc, He also intended healing - total healing of the person. Jesus came into the world to heal. To heal the complete man - his body, mind and soul.

HEALING OF THE CENTURION'S SERVANT

The account of the healing of the centurion's servant is given in Luke 7:1-10 and Mathew 8:5-13. It was when

Jesus entered Capernaum that the centurion approached Jesus. The centurion has a good heart. This fact is evident from the words, "a slave whom he valued highly." He was a man who respected and loved his servant.

He sent some Jewish elders to Jesus, because he was so humble that he considered himself unworthy to approach Jesus. He says to Jesus, "Lord, I am not worthy to have You come under my roof." (Lk. 7:6) The following words of the centurion are the proof of his profound faith. "Therefore, I did not presume to come to You. But only speak the word, and let my servant be healed." (Lk. 7:7)

The Evangelist remarks, "When Jesus heard this, He was amazed at him, and turning to crowd that followed Him, He said, 'I tell you, not even in Israel have I found such faith!'" (Lk. 7:9) And the servant of the centurion was found healed even without a touch of Jesus.

Thus the centurion became a paradigm of faith. His words are repeated even today in our Holy Mass: "Lord, I am not worthy to have you in my home; only say the word, and I shall be healed."

It is because of the centurion's faith that Jesus was able to heal his servant. Similar is the faith and healing of the daughter of the Canaanite women. Jesus tried to discourage her by comparing her and her tribe to "dogs." It was to test her faith that Jesus called her so. But she had an immoveable faith. She had great perseverance. At

31

last, Jesus himself marvels at her faith and grants her the healing she desired.

The centurion and the Canaanite woman are great champions of faith.

A Paralytic Man Healed because of Others' Faith

In the Gospels there is a wonderful example of Jesus healing a man because of the faith of those who brought him to Jesus. St. Mark writes thus, "When He returned to Capernaum after some days, it was reported that He was at home. So many gathered around that there was no longer room for them, not even in front of the door... The some people came, bringing to Him a paralyzed man, carried by four of them. And when they could not bring him to Jesus because of the crowd, they removed the roof above Him. . . . When Jesus saw their faith, He said to the paralytic, 'Son, your sins are forgiven.'" (Mk. 2:1-5)

Here we get an indication that the paralyzed man perhaps had not much faith or expectation to be healed. He was "in sin." But the persons who took initiative to bring him to Jesus had very strong faith. It was because of that faith that they were able to take the risk of removing the roof in order to reach the paralytic down to Jesus. Even today Jesus heals some people because of the faith of others, their friends or relatives.

Another important feature of this healing is that Jesus, first of all, forgives his sins. It indicates that the man had his sins as an obstruction to receive healing.

HEALING AT THE POOL OF BETHESDA

In the Gospel of St. John there is an exclusive incident of Jesus healing a man who had been ill for 38 years (Jn. 5:1-9). The sick man had a sort of faith even before he met Jesus. That was why he waited near the pool. He believed in the healing power of the pool of Bethesda. He had seen many sick people being healed by the healing water in the pool. But he had no one to take him to the pool when the water is stirred up. Thus, after long years, he had been slowly losing his hope.

It was at this juncture that Jesus approaches him. Jesus asks him, "Do you want to be made well? (Jn. 5:6) Have you ever thought why Jesus asked such a question to a man who had been waiting there for such a long time? The man had been in a state of inertia, and his faith and hope had been frozen because he had stayed there for a long time with no one to help him. So what Jesus was trying to do was to stir up the faith and hope in him with a question. He was stirring up the desire of the man to get healed, that desire that had remained frozen. The prerequisites of a person to receive healing are faith, desire and hope. Jesus was rising up these three things in that man. When he has regained his lost optimism and faith, Jesus heals him at once. (Jn. 5:9)

33

JESUS RAISES LAZARUS

Perhaps, the greatest of Jesus' miracles and healings is the raising of Lazarus back to life. The incident is recorded in the Gospel of John Chapter 11. The Chapter begins by these words, "Now a certain man was ill, Lazarus of Bethany." Jesus was informed about the illness of Lazarus. But Jesus replied, "This illness does not lead to death; rather it is for God's glory, so that the Son of God may be glorified through it." (Jn. 11:4)

And Jesus stayed back even for two more days, then He set off to Bethany to meet Lazarus. On the way He revealed that Lazarus has died. When Jesus arrived he found that Lazarus had already been in the tomb for four days. Martha, the sister of Lazarus, came and said that if Jesus had been there her brother would not have died. "Then Jesus told her, 'your brother will rise again." Martha said to Him, "I know that he will rise again in the resurrection on the last day." Jesus said to her, "I am the resurrection and the life. Those who believed in Me, even though they die, will live; and everyone who lives and believed in Me will never die!" (Jn. 11:23-26)

Then there is a touching scene of Jesus weeping at the tomb of Lazarus. (Jn. 11:35) Here, we can perceive the tenderness of the love of Jesus. Jesus, the Son of God; who became son of man for our sake, felt pain with man. He felt the sorrows of mankind. Jesus is a God who feels with man, who weeps with man. His love is divine and human.

"Jesus, then approached the tomb of Lazarus and said, 'Take away the stone.' Martha, the sister of the dead man, said to Him, 'Lord, already there is a stench because he has been dead four days.' Jesus said to her, 'Did I not tell you that if you believed, you would see the glory of God?' So they took away the stone. And Jesus looked upward and said, 'Father, I thank You for having heard Me. I know that You always hear Me, but I have said this for the sake of the crowd standing here, so that they may believe that You sent Me.' When he had said this, he cried with a loud voice, 'Lazarus, come out!' The dead man came out, his hands and feet bound with strips of cloth, and his face wrapped in a cloth." (Jn. 11:39-44)

This incident is unique in history. Four days had passed since the death of Lazarus. His body might have been decayed and stinking. But Jesus with his tremendous power calls him back to life.

JESUS COMMISSION HIS DISCIPLES

After His resurrection, Jesus blessed His disciples and said, "And these sign will accompany those who believe: by using My Name they will cast out demons; they will speak in new tongues; they will pick up snakes in their hands, and if they drink any deadly thing, it will not hurt them; they will lay their hands on the sick, and they will recover." (Mk. 16:16-18) Anyone who believes in Jesus will do works of Jesus. By their faith in Jesus, they will be able to heal the sick. Thus we see in the Acts of the

Apostles, Peter healing a crippled beggar by the powerful Name of Jesus.

A Crippled Beggar Healed by the Name of Jesus

One day Peter and John were going up to the temple at the hour of prayer, at three o'clock in the afternoon. And a man lame from birth was being carried in. People would lay him daily at the gate of the temple called the Beautiful Gate so that he could ask for alms from those entering the temple. When he saw Peter and John about to go into the Temple, he asked them for alms. Peter looked intently at him, as did John, and said, "Look at us!" And he fixed his attention on them, expecting to receive something from them. But Peter said, "I have no silver or gold, but what I have I give you: in the name of Jesus Christ of Nazareth, stand up and walk." And he took him by the right hand and raised him up; and immediately his feet and ankles were made strong. Jumping up, he stood and began to walk, and he entered the temple with them, walking and leaping and praising God. (Acts 3:1-8)

Here we can see the magnificent faith of Peter. He heals the crippled man just by the utterance of a word. The Name of Jesus had become so powerful! The power of that Name worked miracles through his disciples. It is said that even the shadow of St. Peter was powerful enough to heal.

Believe

Jesus said, "Have faith in God. Truly I tell you, if you say to this mountain, 'Be taken up and thrown into the sea!' and if you do not doubt in your heart but believe, what you say will come to pass. It will be done for you. So I tell you, whatever you ask for in prayer, believe that you have received it and it will be yours" (Mk. 11:22-24)

Miracles and healings are done by the power of faith. Jesus says, "Believe what you say will come to pass, it will be done to you." Believe with deep conviction. Ask in prayer with the belief that you have received. This is what we see in the Lazarus incident. Jesus prays to God even before He had raised up Lazarus, "Father, I thank you for having heard me. I know that you always hear me." (Jn. 11:41-42) Jesus is thanking God even before the miracle is realized. He is so certain that it will indeed happen.

DIFFERENT DIMENSIONS OF FAITH HEALING

We have seen different dimensions of faith healing. We have an example in the woman with hemorrhages who had such a tremendous faith that she gained healing by a mere touch on the fringe of the mantle of Jesus. And the Canaanite woman is similar too. Both of them surprised Jesus by the strength of their profound faith.

Another kind of healing is that which is done as in the case of the paralytic. The paralytic is healed not by his own faith, but by the faith of others who brought him to Jesus.

Jesus Desires Gratitude

In the Gospel of Luke, we see an incident of ten lepers. "On the way to Jerusalem, Jesus was going through the region between Samaria and Galilee. As He entered a village, ten lepers approached Him. Keeping their distance, they called out, saying, 'Jesus, Master, have mercy, on us!' When He saw them, He said to them, 'Go and show yourselves to the priests.' And as they went, they were made clean. Then one of them, when he saw that he was healed, turned back, praising God with a loud voice. He prostrated himself at Jesus' feet and thanked Him. And he was a Samaritan. Jesus said, "Were not ten made clean? But the other nine, where are they? Has none of them returned to give praise to God except this foreigner?" (Lk. 17:11-18) The last words express the pain of Jesus at the ingratitude of the nine lepers who did not even think to come back and thank Jesus, "were not ten made clean? But the other nine, where are they?"

This instance clearly indicates that even Jesus desires the gratitude of man. One must be thankful to God for the blessings one has received, whether it be healing or not, give praise to God for the healing.

Often we tend to forget the Healer is God when we receive some healing. Remember that we have obligation to praise and thank God and to live a life of praise. We must lead a holy life pleasing to God thereafter. That is the way we should express our gratitude to God!

CHAPTER 5
HEALING OF THE TOTAL PERSON

Often people seek only the healing of the body. But man is a combination of mind, soul and body. According to modern medical science, most of the physical ailments are caused by tensions, worries and hatred. Tensions and anxieties can be the cause of cancer. We have experienced more than once that tensions can cause headaches and stomach disorders. They are called psychosomatic sickness.

Today's world is a busy world. Life has become hastier than ever. The more busy life becomes, the more tensions man gets. The more desires man has, the more unsatisfied he be comes. Man runs after so many things, but in the end he realizes that his heart is empty in spite of every worldly thing he has gained. Remember the words of St. Augustine, "O God, You have created us for Yourself. Our heart will not find rest until they rest in You." Our hearts are created for God. Our souls are created in the image and likeness of God. So, they will never find true rest and happiness until they rest in God. St. Augustine was a worldly young man from Tagaste in Africa. He had a great thirst for knowledge and carnal pleasures. So, he went in search of all these kinds of pleasures, he lived with all kinds of worldly pleasures. But in the end he felt very much dissatisfied.

Once, he heard a voice saying to him, "Take and read." He took it as a command from Heaven to read the Scriptures and he read the passage, "The night is far gone, the day is near. Let us then lay aside the works of darkness and put on the armor of light. Let us live honorably as in the day, not in reveling and darkness, not in debauchery and licentiousness, not in quarrelling and jealousy. Instead, put on the Lord Jesus Christ, and make no provisions for the flesh, to gratify its desires." (Ro. 13:12-14) St. Augustine at once obeyed the command of God. He abandoned every evil desires and dedicated himself to God. He experiences the joy of living with God. Thus he exclaimed, "O Ever-old and Ever-new Beauty, late have I loved you!." This moving story is narrated in his famous autobiography named, "Confessions."

The life of St. Augustine is and example and model to modern man who is entangled in sin and pursuit after worldly pleasures. St. Augustine is typical to modern man in two ways. One is his thirst for knowledge. Today, man is after newer knowledge and technology. Every day there are new discoveries. Science is rapidly progressing.

Computers and super-computers emerge. Cloning. Man is never satisfied with knowledge.

Another is his desire for bodily pleasures. Modern man is obsessed with sexual pleasures. Morality is cast away. Everywhere we can see free sex and pornography in films, on the Internet, etc. But he is never satisfied. There is only one answer for it, "O God, you have created our hearts for Yourself. They will not find rest until they rest in You."

In the Twentieth Century we have an example similar to St. Augustine. It is Thomas Merton, the famous American mystic. He too had lived a wayward and worldly life in his teens and youth. But finally getting disgusted with the meaningless pleasures of the world, he left the world and entered a Trappist monastery named Gethsemane in Kentucky. In his renowned autobiography, "Seven Story Mountain," he depicts his spiritual transformation.

You might have read about Marilyn Monroe, an actress renowned for her charm and beauty. She had millions of admirers around the world. She had immense wealth and every kind of fortune a woman can get in this world. But she committed suicide because she was depressed and was very lonely within.

"If you gain the whole world, but lose your soul, what is the use?" St. Francis Xavier, a brilliant and ambitions student at the University of Paris heard these words. St. Ignatius of Loyola uttered these words into his ears. It touched St. Francis and transformed him. He abandoned his academic career and left Europe as a missionary. He came to India and Japan and preached the Gospel. He baptized thousands of people. Today he is the co-patron of the missions, together with St. Therese of the Child Jesus.

The world is in a rush after worldly pleasures and ambitions. They never realize that the gaining of every riches in the world is of no use if one loses his soul.

Now, we have seen that mental disorders and tensions can be the cause of bodily sicknesses. Even deeper is the part played by sin in making man sick. Every sickness came into the world because of sin. In the Garden of Eden, before the original sin, man was extremely happy and healthy. He never had any illness. He was wholesome but sin brought disorders into man. It destroyed his soul. The disorders of the soul and loss of God's grace made man vulnerable to all kinds of illness. Jesus says to the man whom he healed at the pool of Bethesda, "See, you have been made well. Do not sin anymore, so that nothing worse happens to you." (Jn. 5:14) Here, Jesus clearly says that sin was the cause of his illness.

THE TOTAL PERSON THERAPY OF JESUS

As man is a combination of soul, mind and body, he is to be healed in all three realms in order to become wholesome. Sin is the sickness of the soul. The mind has mental and emotional disorders. And the body has physical illness.

I will speak of each, and also describe the different medicines for each.

A. The Sickness of the Soul

Sin is actually the illness of the soul. When God created man, he had sanctifying grace, which could be compared to the immunity power against sin. He enjoyed the company of God. He was always happy because he had a happy and healthy soul in which God dwelt. He was in peace with the nature. The wild animals obeyed him. Every tree bore fruits for him. The moment he disobeyed God and committed sin; he lost the company and union with God. His soul became unhealthy fear and guilt-consciousness entered into his soul. He became vulnerable to sin. Thereafter, man began to be born with the stain of original sin.

This state is depicted by St. Paul in his letter to the Romans. "For I know that nothing good dwells in me, that is, in my flesh. I can will what is right, but I cannot do it; for I do not do the good I want, but the evil I do not want. Now if I do what I do not want, it is no longer I that do it but sin that dwells in me." (Ro. 7:16-20) We have also experienced this miserable plight in our life, a number of times, often we have stood helpless before an urge within us to do wrong, rather than right. This is the impact of the original sin. It is a wound, a scar of the old wound in our soul.

1. Prayer Medicine

Repentance is the Prayer medicine to the sickness of the soul. Repentance is the feeling of grief or regret over the sin remitted. King David, a favorite of God, was actually a shepherd boy. But God in His abundant mercy, made him the king if Israel. But he succumbed to his impure passions and committed adultery with the wife of his servant Uriah. Moreover, he killed Uriah in treachery in order to hide his sin. This angered God. God sent his prophet Nathan to chide David. David was heartbroken. He repented of his sin. Thus he wrote the famous Psalm of repentance, "Have mercy on me, O God, according to Your steadfast love; according to Your abundant mercy. Blot out my transgressions. Wash me thoroughly from my iniquity and cleanse me from my sin." (Ps. 51:1-2)

True repentance is born out of love of God. It is a feeling and awareness that I have caused pain to God who has loved me so much.

Jesus has loved us to the point of shedding His blood for us and dying. He has died for us. Neither our father nor our mother has died for us. Our brother or sister, or our girlfriend or boyfriend, have not died for us. But Jesus has died for us on the cross. When we remember this fact, our hearts will break into tears, over the pain we have caused Him by our sins. Every sin of ours is a wound upon the sacred body of Jesus.

In his autography titled, "Treasure in Clay," Archbishop Fulton J. Sheen writes, "The crucifix is my autobiography. It is not something that I narrate to you, but something that I read myself. I see my swelling pride in His crown of thorns, and my greedy ventures to grab the earthly vanities in His pierced palms. In His wounded feet I recognize my evasions from my pastoral responsibilities; my wasted love in His broken heart, and my impure thoughts in that piece of flesh that hangs from His side like some scarlet rag. And whenever I go through the pages of this autobiography my heart bursts into tears upon the ungrateful deeds I, His adopted friend, have done against the Divine Friend!"

2. Sacramental Medicine

Confession and reconciliation are the sacramental medicine for the sickness of the soul. A sacrament is the visible sign of an invisible grace. Confession is the act of disclosing our sin to a priest who is the representative of Christ. It is not the priest who absolves the sin, but Christ who is hidden behind. Jesus himself has imparted the authority to forgive sins to his disciples. After His resurrection, Jesus appeared to His disciples and said,

"'Peace be with you. As the Father has sent me, so I send you.' When He said this, He breathed on them and said to them, 'Receive the Holy Spirit. If you forgive the sins of any, they are forgiven them. If you retain the sins of any, they are retained.'" (Jn. 20:21-23)

Jesus gave this authority to the apostles. By tradition, this authority is passed down to the bishops of the Catholic Church, for they are the successors of the apostles. As the vicars of the bishops, priests enjoy this power of absolution. So, it is very important to confess our sins to a priest in order to receive absolution.

Reconciliation is also very important. Broken relationships are to be corrected and healed. Grace will not flow through broken relationships. Take the example of the electric circuit. The power supply will be blocked if the wire is broken anywhere. Similarly, when our relationship with God and our fellow beings are broken, the flow of grace will be blocked. In order to reset the flow the wire should be rejoined.

Once, during one of my retreats in Kerala, there attended a man with a dagger at his waist. He had come there to kill his rival, who was also attending the retreat. This rival had killed his only son some years back. The class on forgiveness and reconciliation was going on. I spoke about the forgiving love of Jesus, who forgave and prayed for His enemies. The word of God touched him like a lightning. He got up from his seat at once, threw the dagger at the altar with a loud scream, and he came to his rival, knelt down before him and begged his forgiveness. Being profoundly moved, the rival also began to weep. The whole congregation wept at this touching act of reconciliation.

Jesus says in the Gospel, "So when you are offering your gift at the altar, if you remember that your brother or sister has something against you, leave your gift there before the altar and go; first be reconciled to your brother or sister, and then come and offer your gift." (Mt. 5:23-24)

God will not accept our gifts if we are still keeping grudge against our fellow beings. God is our Father. All human beings are his children. So, they are our brothers and sisters too. That is why reconciliation is necessary. It is the healing of relationships.

B. Sickness of the Mind

The human mind is also vulnerable to illness and disorders. It is caused by emotional disorders. They have psychological reasons. Human mind is divided into three parts: the conscious mind, subconscious mind and unconscious mind. 5/9ths of our mind is the unconscious mind, 3/9ths belongs to subconscious region and only 1/9th is our conscious mind.

Whatever enters into our mind remains in the conscious mind for a while and then it sinks into the subconscious mental region. Ultimately in the long run it is buried in the unconscious mind. But the experiences and memories both in the subconscious and unconscious regions of our mind can affect our behavior positively or negatively, depending upon their nature.

Here lies the reason for our occasional strange behaviors, which even puzzle us. Some kinds of fears, inhibitions, phobias, anxieties and so on have their roots in the subconscious recesses of our mind. The negative experience we had while were in our mother's womb could negatively affect our life. Even the thoughts, fears, anxieties and hatred of the pregnant mother can affect the child in the womb in its later life. The child, whom his parents had planned to abort while it was still in the womb, will have a feeling of unwantedness in its later life. In the lives of some, there are unexplainable fears and anxieties, various kinds of phobias, as the psychologists would call them. Some people have irrational fear of insects, spiders, cockroaches, etc. Some have fear of darkness. Another ones fear narrow places, water, lightning and thunder, etc.

Such fears may have their root in its mother during her pregnancy period. While pregnant, she might have got frightened at the sight of in-sects or darkness. The incident of John the Baptist in the Bible gives testimony how the feeling of the mother can affect the body in the womb. When Mary came and greeted the pregnant Elizabeth, John was just six months old in his mother's womb. Still, he was overjoyed. As the Bible says, "The child in the womb leaped with joy." (Lk. 1:44) The joy of his mother affected the child. Similarly, bad incidents and feelings that affect the mother negatively, can affect the child negatively too.

1. Prayer Medicine

Inner healing is the prayer medicine for the sickness of the mind. Inner healing is the healing of memories and the effects of negative experiences in one's mind. Jesus can bring inner healing. Because "Jesus Christ is the same yesterday, today and tomorrow" (Heb. 13:8) our past is not past for Jesus. He has authority over past and future. He has no past, no future. He is eternal! He is always in the present. He is present in past and future. So, He can enter into our past; heal our memories, even if they are rooted in the unconscious region of our mind.

We must invite Jesus into our memories. We should ask Him to enter into our past and heal our negative experiences of our past. Implore Him to touch our inner wounds, the bitter experience we had while we were still in our mother's womb or those we had while we were still babies. His touch will certainly heal us.

Because Jesus has authority over the past, he has power over our mind and our negative feelings. During every retreat, many are healed of their bad habits, their anger, hatred, unforgiveness, uncontrolled sexuality, etc. Jesus can transform these internal handicaps to their greater good. There are many examples in the Bible and history of the church, of persons whose weakness were transformed by God as their power and merit. St. Mary Magdalene, St. Paul, St. Augustine are a few examples.

Just take the example of St. Mary Magdalene. She was a sinner and an adulteress. She was a woman thirsting for love. The love perverted made her commit adultery. When the love of Jesus healed her inner wounds, all her capability to love became holy. Thus, she became one of the greatest lovers of God. Similar is the case of St. Augustine. He indulged in carnal passion during his earlier days. But when the love of Jesus touched him and healed his mind from the stains of the past, he exclaimed with holy and ardent love for God, "Late have I loved you, O Ever-old and Ever-new Beauty!"

Invite Jesus into your past memories, imagine that Jesus is touching you. Tell Him when He comes before you, like the leper in the Gospel, "If you choose Lord, you can make me clean." (Mk. 1:40)

2. Sacramental Medicine

Confession and the reception of the Holy communion can heal your mind. Through confession, we have both an effect of the relief of the mind, and the flow of God's grace. By the reception of the Holy Communion, we are actually receiving Jesus Christ into our heart. The grace that is showered upon us while receiving the Holy Eucharist has great healing effect.

3. Natural Medicine

Counseling is the natural medicine. What I mean here is the spiritual counseling using the gifts of the Holy Spirit. The Holy Spirit unveils to us the wounds in our memory during the counseling. The Holy Spirit gives us the wisdom through which the person's mind could be healed.

C. Sickness of the Body

Sin and its effects cause 87 percent of bodily sicknesses. Accidents, germs, viruses and bacteria cause the remaining 13 percent.

1. Prayer Medicine

Faith Healing is the prayer medicine to physical illness. Jesus gives the authority and power to his disciples to heal. "They [those who believe] will lay their hands on the sick, and they will recover." (Mk. 16:18) We have numerous instances in the Holy Scriptures of the healing by faith.

2. Sacrament Medicine

Anointing with the holy oil is the sacrament medicine to the physical illness. Its biblical basis is in the Gospel of Mark. "They cast out many demons, and anointed with oil any who were sick, and cured them." (Mk. 6:13) In the letter of James we can see a clear reference and exhortation to use oil to cure the sick. "Are any among you suffering? They should pray. Are any among you sick? They should call for the elders and have them pray over them, anointing them with oil in the name of the Lord. The prayer of faith will save the sick, and the Lord will raise them up." (Jas. 5:13-15)

But we should not avoid the oil of natural medicines and doctors because the word of God says, "Honor physicians for their services, for the Lord created them; for their gift of healing comes from the Most High (Sir. 38:1-2). The book of Wisdom says, "For neither herb nor poultice cured them, but it was Your word, O Lord, that heals all people." (Wis. 16:12)

CHAPTER 6
SIMPLE FAITH AND THE POWER OF PRAYER

Once, an acrobat was exhibiting his balance and skill by walking upon a rope tied across the great Niagara Falls. Thousands of people gathered there watched, holding their breaths. This man succeeded to walk across the great waterfalls on a rope. There was a loud applause of wonder. Then the acrobat asked them whether any mother there would hand over her child to him so that he could carry the child with him as walks across the waterfalls the next time. Suddenly, a silence of awe fell upon the scene. Nobody dared. Mothers hugged their children tightly. The acrobat kept watch. At last a little boy came forward with a smile. Without any fear or hesitation, the child climbed upon the shoulders of the acrobat. As everybody stood spellbound, the acrobat carried the boy safely across the waterfalls. Amazed the people asked who the fearless child was. The boy answered with a smile, "Why should I be afraid when I am sitting on the shoulders of my father?"

This is the attitude of one who has faith and trust in God. He is confident that he is safe upon the shoulders of God who is a loving Father. The Father cares for him. The Father who loves him is thoughtful of him. He is confident.

Jesus taught us to call God, "Our Father." Jesus gave us the "Abba" concept. "Abba" is the term used to show the close intimacy of a child to its father. It is similar to our "Dad." Jesus intended that we must have a deeply personal relationship with the Father. This trust and confidence in God is the essence of faith. It is the mentality of a child holding the finger of God.

Great saints were people with simple faith. St. Theresa of the Child Jesus, one of the greatest saints of the modern times, had simple faith and childlike confidence in God. St. Francis of Assisi looked upon God as a caring Father. He advised his disciples to live with complete abandonment into the providence of God. The faith of Abraham, the father of the faithful, was essentially simple. It was a complete trust in God. God asked him to abandon his homeland and go to a land shown by God. He obeyed it in faith. Then God commanded him to offer the life of his only child Isaac in sacrifice to God. Without a word of rebellion he obeyed. That is the power of simple and absolute faith.

Today's world is a complicated one. Many complicated teachings and branches of knowledge have made things complicated. But essentially, faith is simple. The more our faith becomes complicated, the more doubtful our minds will become. As we learn more and more, we will acquire a kind of intellectual pride. We start to believe that we know many things; and we will spurn simple faith and trust in God. That is a tragedy in today's world. We became immersed in scientific knowledge and psychological knowledge. Thus we make God a mere object. In fact, God is a person to be loved, not an object to be studied or comprehended. Faith is not faith if it demands full knowledge and understanding with proofs as the scientists do.

Faith is trusting in the things said and done by God just because we believe in Him, that He is God and so He will never lie. The Bible is the words of Jesus Christ. Jesus Christ is God. And so, He will never tell a lie. So, the Bible is all truth. We should never doubt what God has promised. If we acquire such a faith, a faith without doubt, we will be able to perform miracles. Such was the faith of the saints. They trusted the Word of God. They believed whatever God has said, without doubt. So, God worked wonders for them.

PRAYER

"Prayer is a loving conversation with God who we know loves us," says St. Teresa of Avila, the great saint. "Prayer is a loving gaze towards heaven," said St. Therese the Little Flower. Prayer is essentially a friendly talk with God. It is an act of friendly relationship. For prayer, we must have faith that God exists and that He loves us. We will not get wearied or bored when we spend our time with a person whom we love. Speak to God just as you would speak to your intimate friend. Say everything to him – your dreams, your ambitions, your worries, your fears, your joys and your sorrows.

God does not care for the beauty of language, the correctness of your grammar, figures of speech and so on. He tests your heart, your sincerity, your faithfulness, and your love. The heart is what matters, not words.

It is the same thing that is essential when we present our offering before the Lord. Jesus teaches this through the parable of the widow who offered two copper coins. Jesus was watching everybody who was casting his or her offerings into the temple-offering box. All of them were offering from their abundance, what came as surplus? But the widow offered whatever she had. Her heart was with her offering. That was why Jesus valued it above all. Similarly, it is our heart that matters in prayer. Not our bombastic words.

Faith, hope and love – the three theological virtues of Christian life are what are essential for prayer. Believe and trust in God. Love Him deeply, and put your hope in God. Then life is indeed beautiful!

GOD BLESS YOU

Facts on the life of Fr. Bill

Date of Birth: February 23, 1928

Ordination: October 12, 1958

'Divine touch' 1976

Popular mission retreats in India 1981 – 1992

Total number popular mission (approx.) 1,500

To Africa 1992

Countries visited worldwide 72

Total number of retreats worldwide (approx.) 4,600

Total number of attendees worldwide (approx.) more than 5 billion

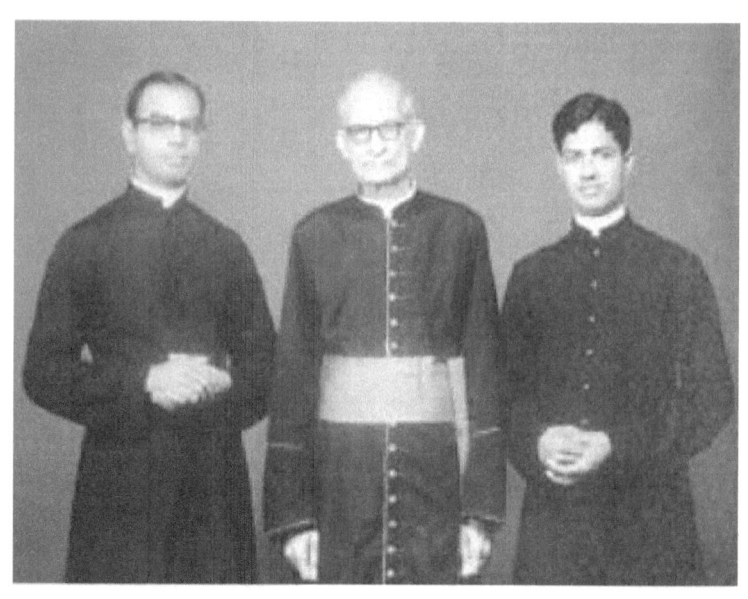

Fr. Bill newly ordained

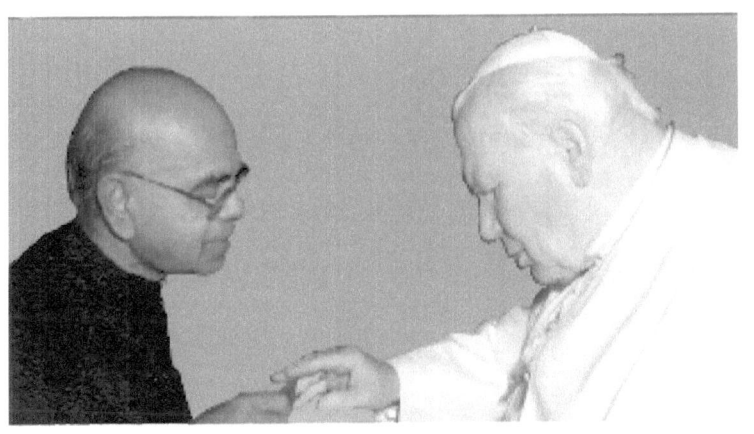

Go out and teach the whole world

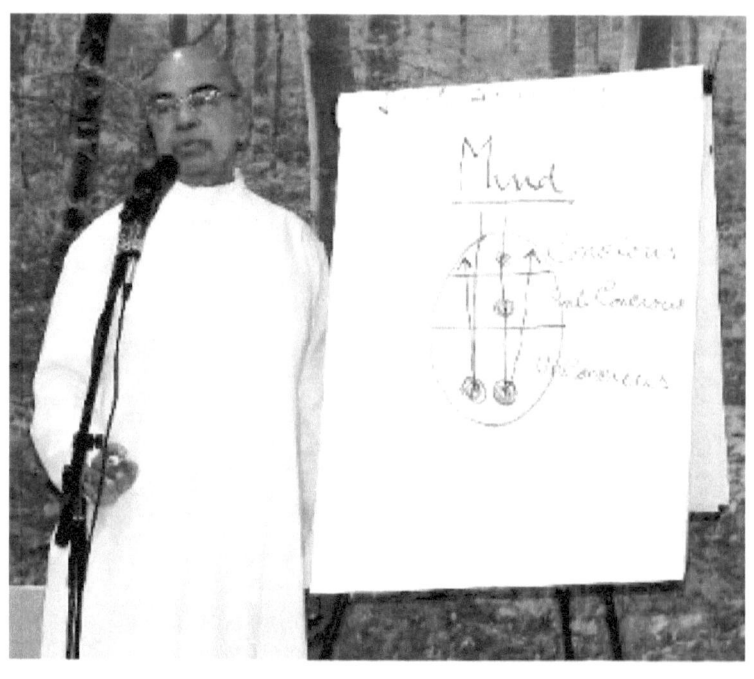

Healing the conscious, subconscious, and unconcious
mind

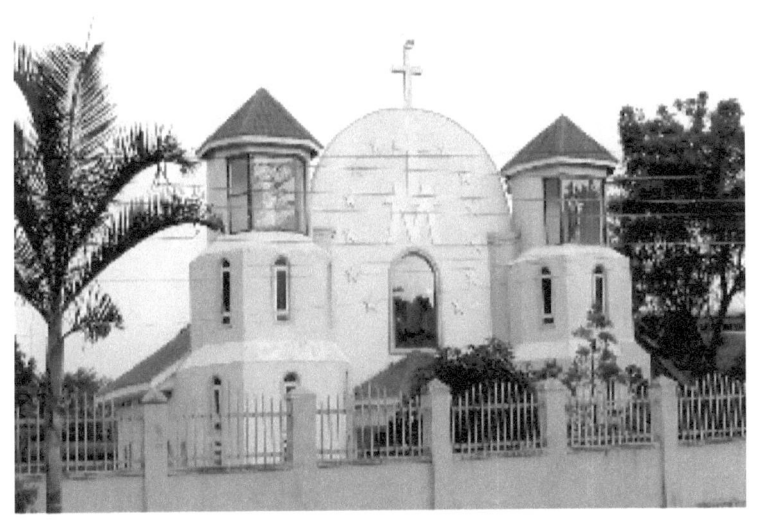

Miraculous Medal Shrine in Entebbe Uganda

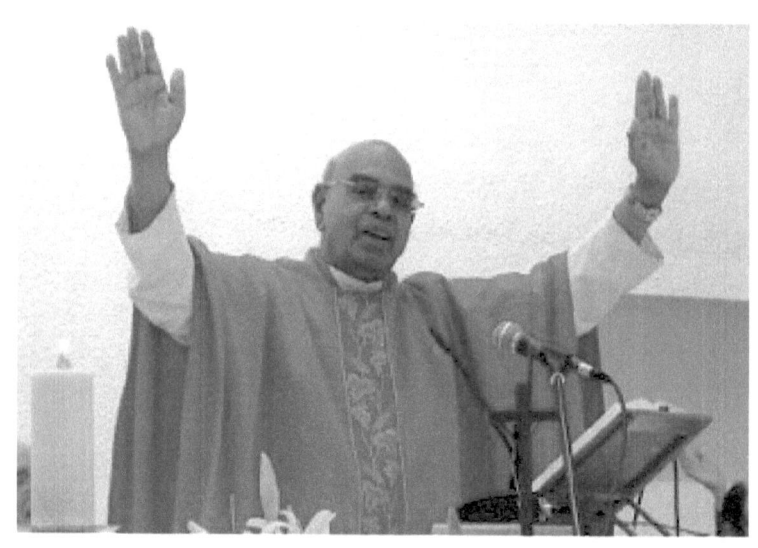

Preaching in Ireland

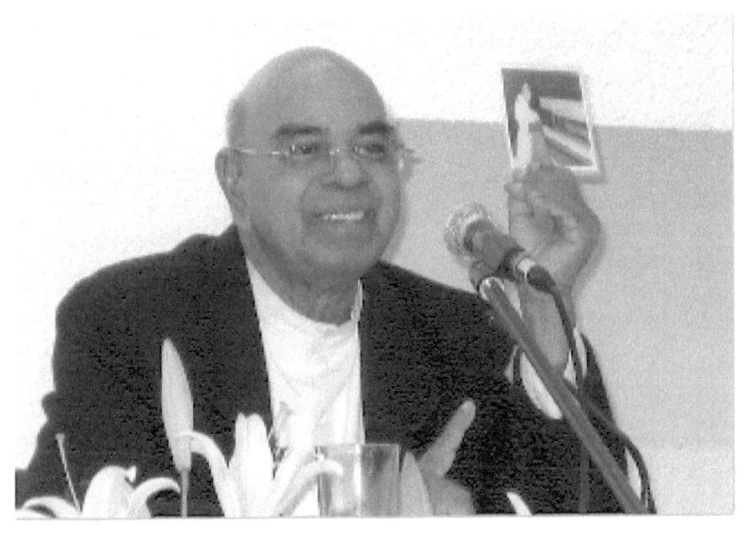

When you become a Saint the Pope will come and Pray

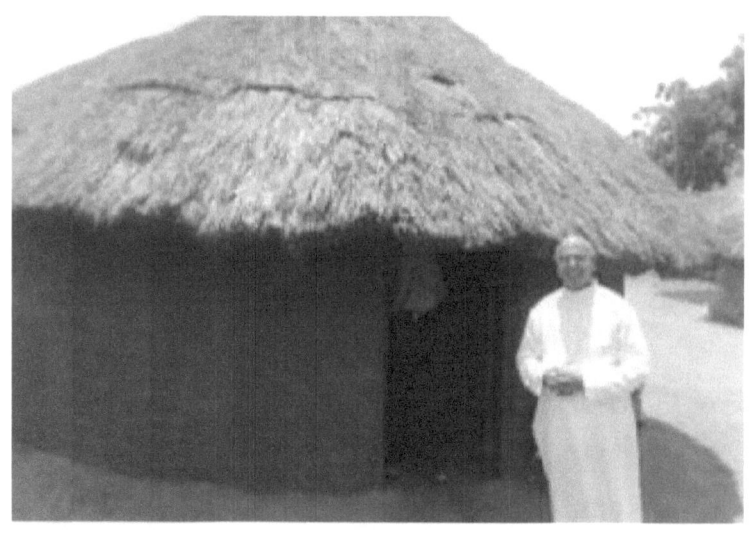

Fr. Bill (March 2008)

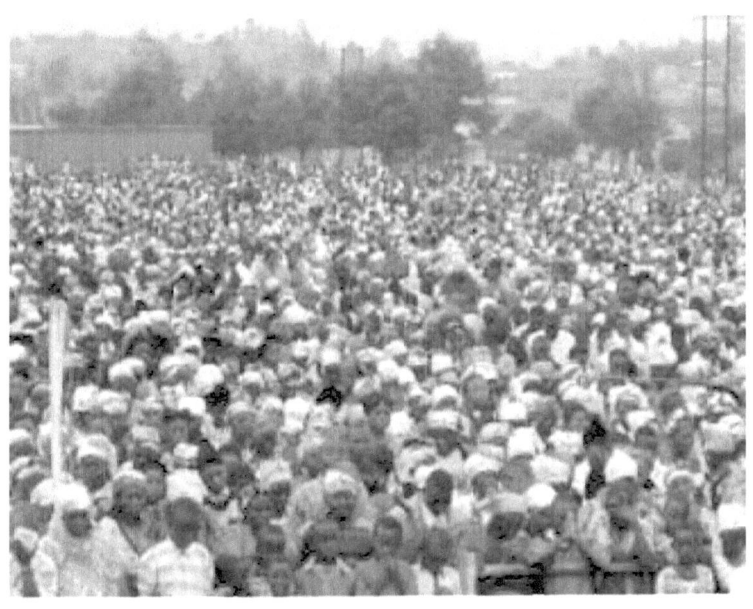

Fr. Bill preaching to a large cowd in Africa

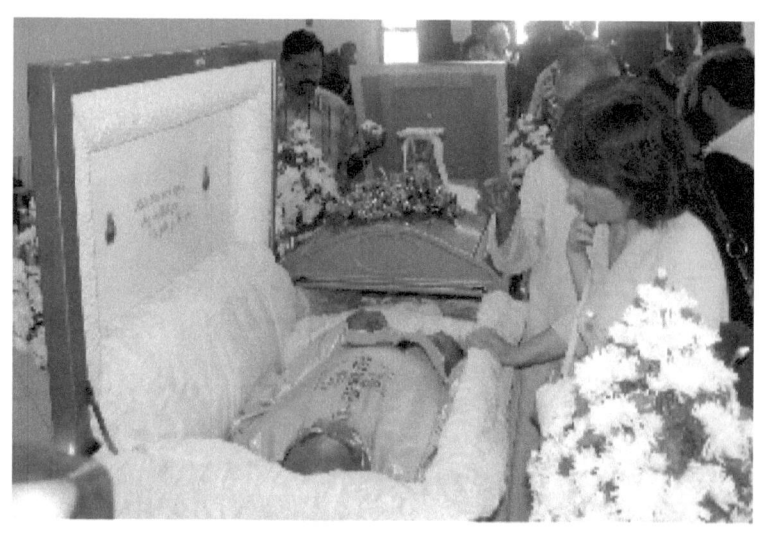

10's of thousands mourn the passing of our Beloved
Fr.Bill.